What Every Woman Should Have

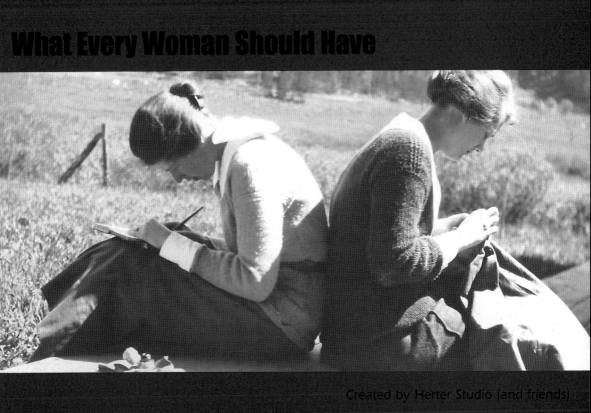

Created by Herter Studio (and friends)

Ten Speed Press
Berkeley/Toronto

every woman

should have

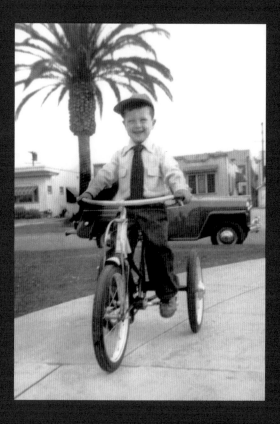

one old boyfriend you can imagine going back to

and one who reminds you of how far you've come.

enough money within your control to
move out and rent a place on your own
even if you never want to

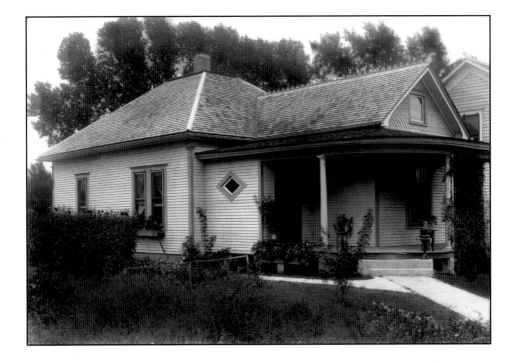

or need to.

something
perfect
to
wear
if
the
employer
or
man of your dreams
wants
to
see
you

in an hour.

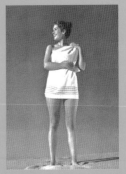

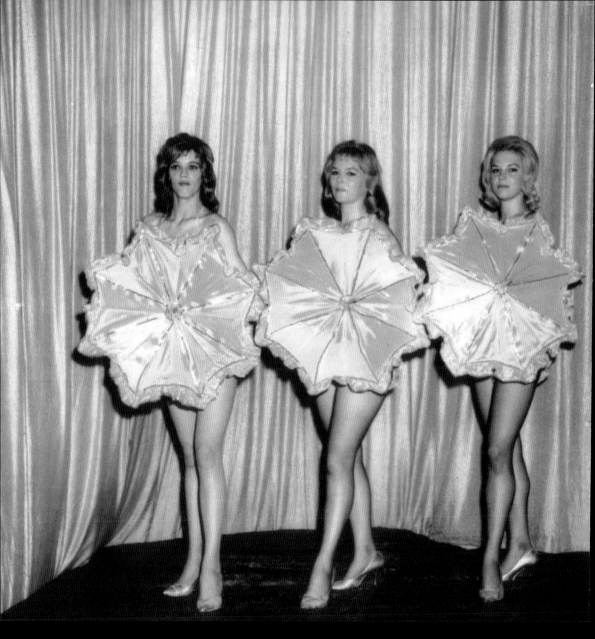

a purse,

a suitcase,

and an umbrella

you're

not ashamed

to be seen carrying.

a youth you're content to move beyond.

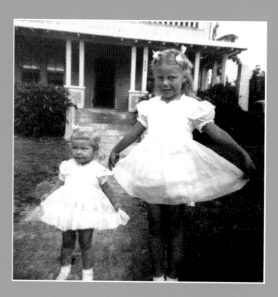

a past **juicy** enough
that you are looking forward to retelling it in your old age.

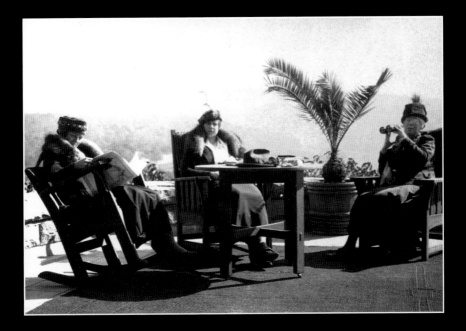

the realization that you are going to have an old age

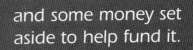

and some money set
aside to help fund it.

a set of screwdrivers

a cordless drill

a black lace bra

one friend who always makes you laugh

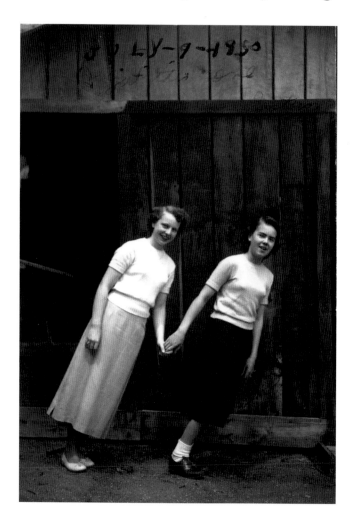

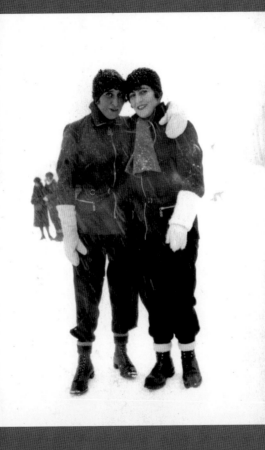

and one who lets you cry.

a good piece of furniture

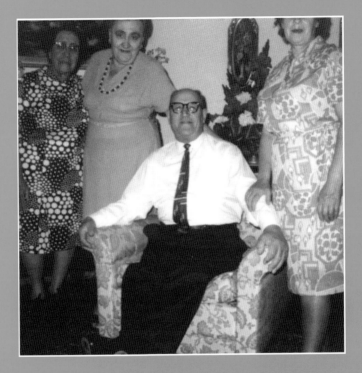

not previously owned by anyone else in your family.

8 matching plates,

wineglasses with stems ,

and a recipe for a meal

that will make your guests

f e e l   h o n o r e d .

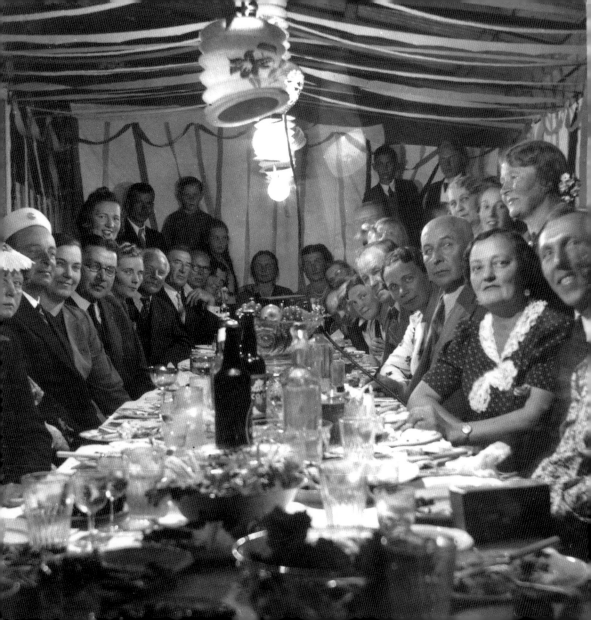

a resume that is not even the slightest bit padded.

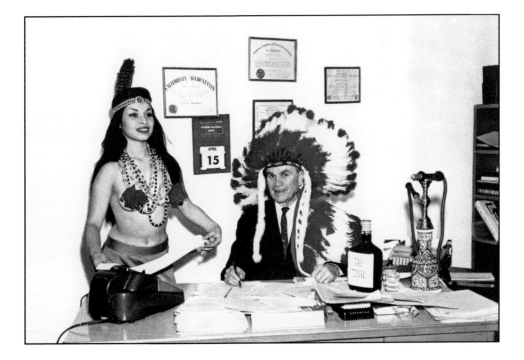

a feeling of control over your destiny.

a skin care regime,

an exercise routine,

and a plan

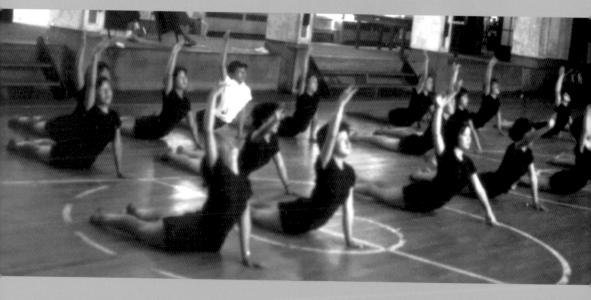

for dealing with those

few other facets of life

that don't get better.

a *solid start on*:

a satisfying career

a satisfying relationship

and all those other

facets *of* life

that

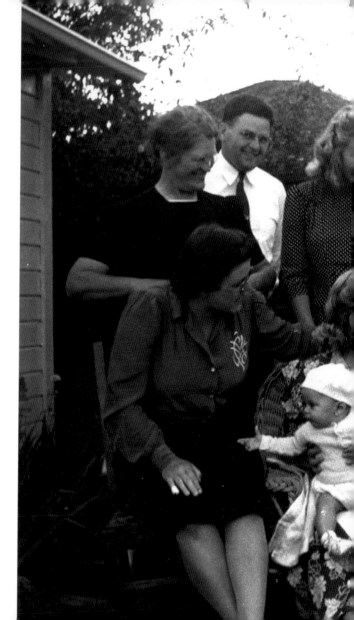

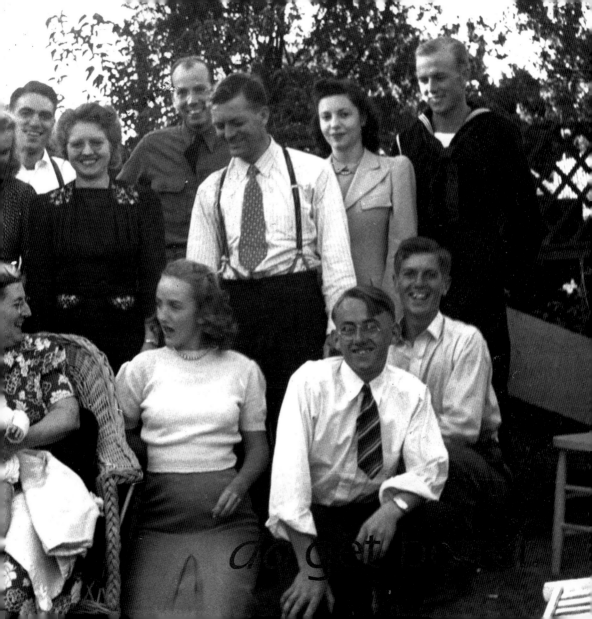

every woman

should know

how to fall in love without losing yourself.

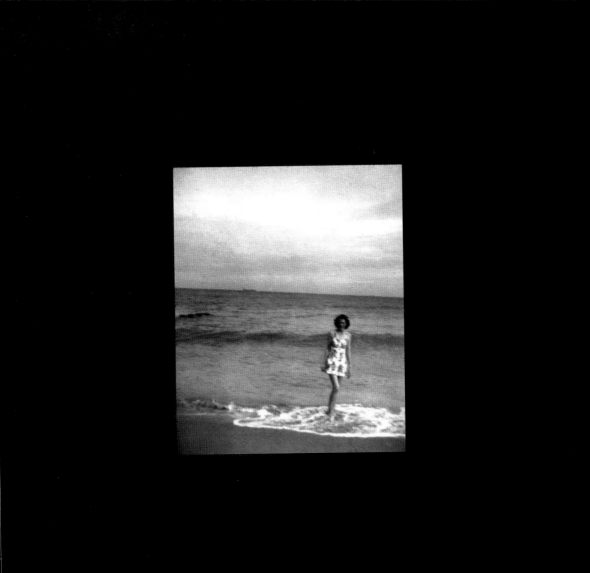

how you feel about having

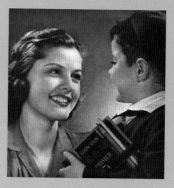

kids.

how to

quit a job,

break up with a man,

and confront a friend without ruining the friendship.

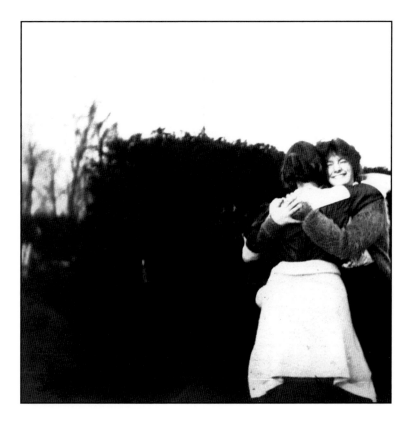

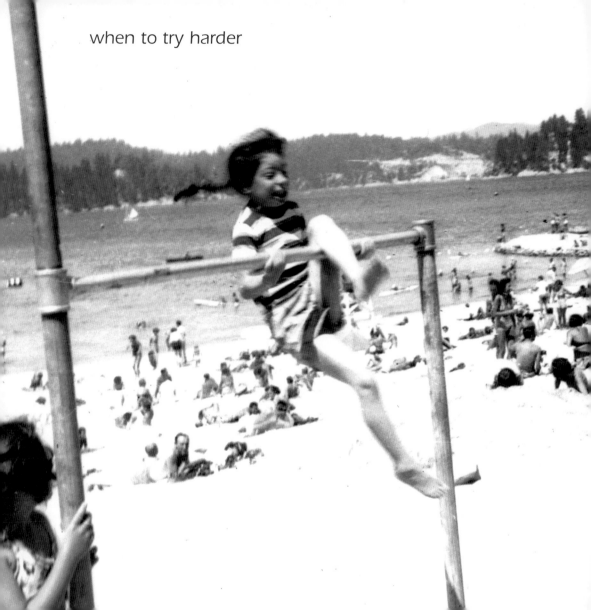

when to try harder

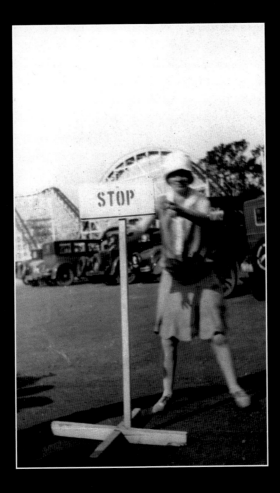

and when to walk away.

how to kiss

a man

in a way

that communicates

p e r f e c t l y

what you

would

and wouldn't

like to happen

next.

how to ask for what you want
in a way that makes it most likely

you'll get it.

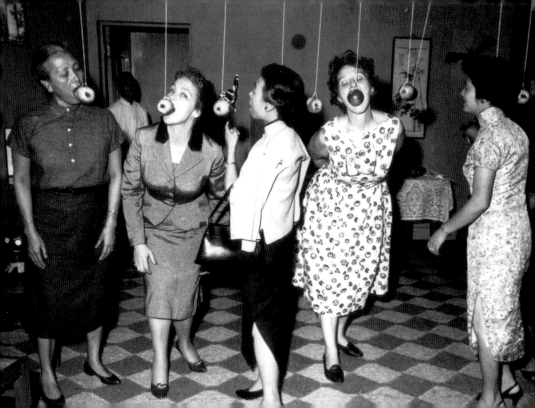

how to have a good time at a party

you'd never choose to attend.

that you can't change

the width of your hips,

the length of your calves,

or the nature of your

parents.

that your childhood may not have been perfect

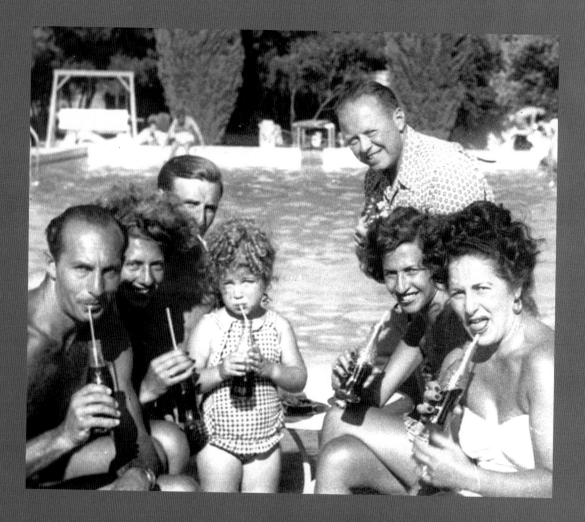

but it's over.

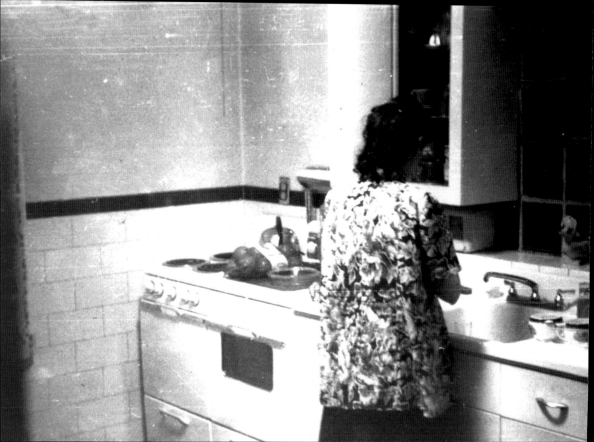

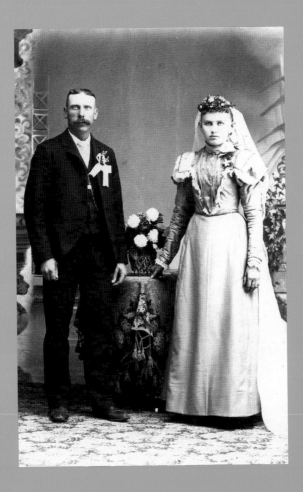

or money.

how to live alone

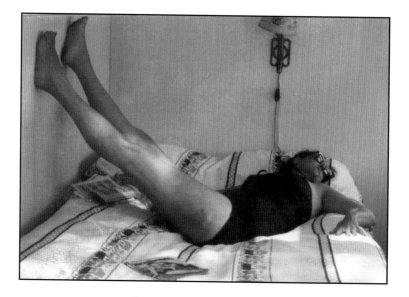

even if you don't like it.

who you **can** trust

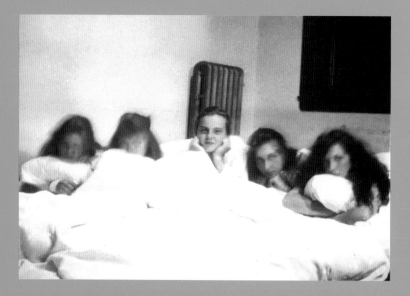

who you **can't**

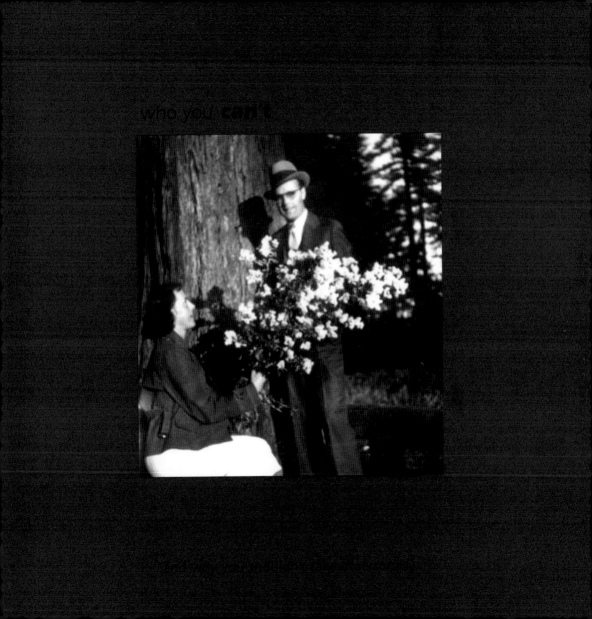

where to go

be it your best friend's kitchen table
or a charming inn hidden in the woods

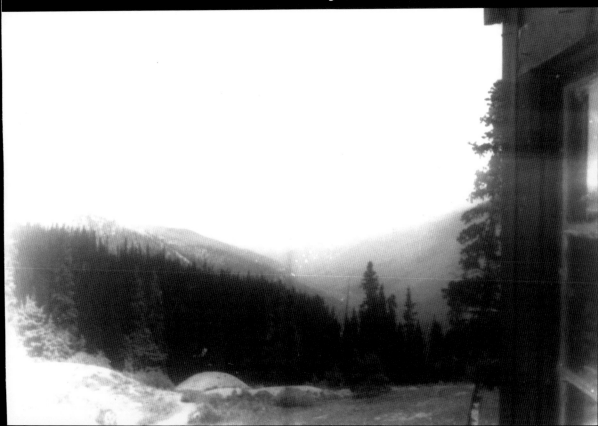

when your soul needs soothing.

what you can and can't accomplish in

a day

a month

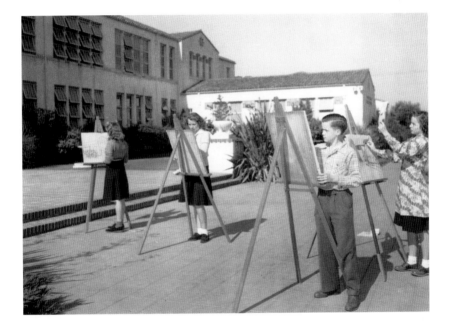

a year.

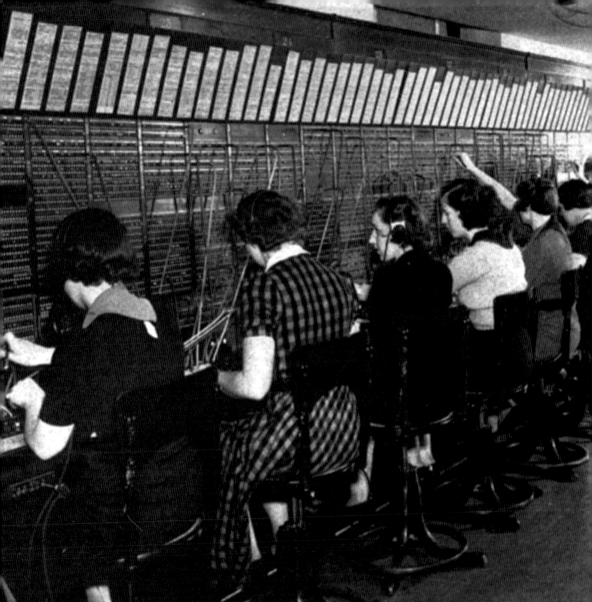

why they say

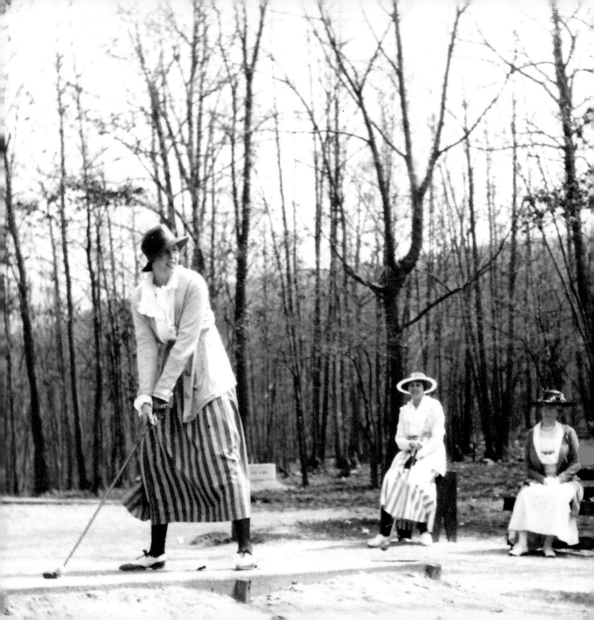

life begins

right now.

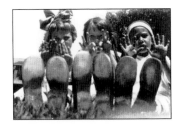

Our gratitude to Kirsty Melville at Ten Speed, for seeing what we saw and going for it, and to Andrew Clarke and Laura Lovett for their expert technical guidance and great patience.

A Note from Herter Studio:
As of this printing, the authorship of What Every Woman Should Have remains
a mystery. You can find the poem on many websites, some of which offer it in
electronic greeting card form. Herter Studio has made all reasonable efforts to
track down the copyright holder of the text, and is prepared to pay fair and reasonable usage fees to the now-unknown original creator for text or photographs
used here without prior consent. The images were sourced from flea markets,
private collectors, family albums, and image banks as follows: Photographs pp.
6, 9, 12, 14, 20-21, 25, 29-30, 43, 48, 56, 58-59, 63, 71 reprinted courtesy of
A Thousand Words, San Francisco. Photographs pp. 23, 32-33, 37, 42, 47, 52, 54-
55, 61 reprinted courtesy of David Murray. Photographs pp. 3, 15, 17, 41, 66
reprinted courtesy of Herter Studio. Photographs cover, pp. 1, 7, 11, 27, 38, 64
© 2001-2002 www.arttoday.com.

Ten Speed Press
Box 7123
Berkeley, California 94707
www.tenspeed.com

A Kirsty Melville Book

Herter Studio
432 Elizabeth Street
San Francisco, CA 94114
www.herterstudio.com

Distributed in Australia by Allen
& Unwin, in Canada by Ten Speed
Press Canada, in New Zealand by
Southern Publishers Group, in
South Africa by Real Books, in
Southeast Asia by Berkeley Books,
and in the United Kingdom and
Europe by Airlift Book Company.

Library of Congress Cataloging-in-
Publication Data on file with
publisher.

Printed in China.
First printing, 2002

1 2 3 4 5 6 7 — 07 06 05 04 03 02